Elf-help for the Mother-to-Be

Elf-help for the Mother-to-Be

written by
Claudia Bollwinkel

illustrated by
R.W. Alley

ONE
CARING
PLACE
Abbey Press

Text © 2006 by Claudia Bollwinkel
Illustrations © 2006 by Saint Meinrad Archabbey
Published by One Caring Place
Abbey Press
St. Meinrad, Indiana 47577

Library of Congress Catalog Number
2006902796

ISBN 0-87029-400-8

Printed in the United States of America

Foreword

You are a mother-to-be! A new life begins—your baby's new life, and also your new life.

The wonder of this occasion easily throws your life out of balance. There are so many changes. Changes in your body. Changes in your public and family roles. There are also worries about living arrangements and the finances of parenthood.

Elf-help for the Mother-to-Be provides hints on how to enjoy the precious time of pregnancy and how to let go of your worries. *Elf-help* helps you ease into motherhood and enjoy your new baby.

A happy mother-to-be knows how to let go. What you need most now is trust—trust in yourself, in your child, in your partner, in the future, and in God. God wanted this miracle to happen. Now let God do the work!

1.

Thank God! You are being given a brand new love—the love for your unborn child now growing like a beautiful flower.

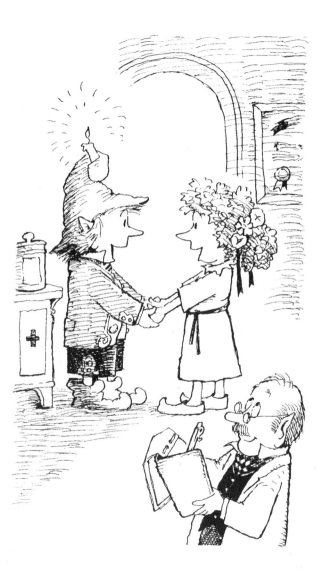

2.

Pay attention to the many changes occurring both within you and outside of you.

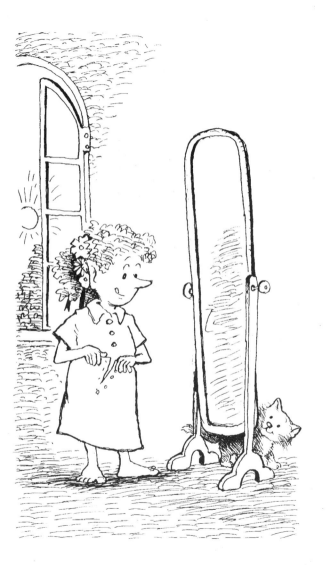

3.

Share your happiness with other people. A child is a gift to the whole world.

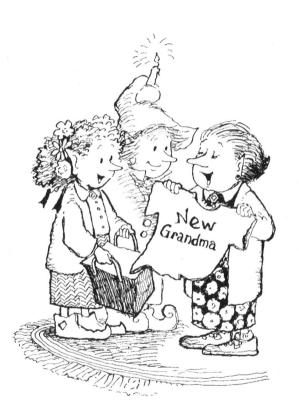

4.

Accept your condition.
Your child is growing
and wants your attention.

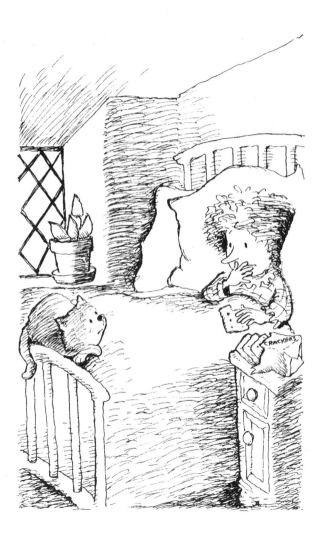

5.

Sleep a lot. You and your child grow closer while sleeping.

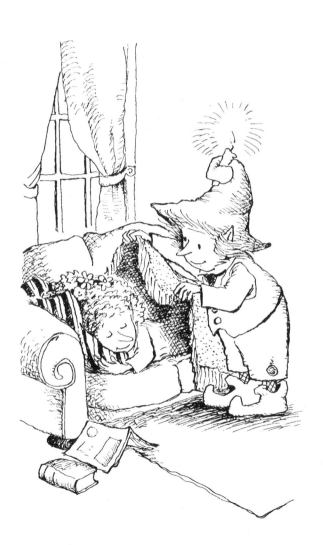

6.

Spend more time alone.
You need silence
to hear yourself.

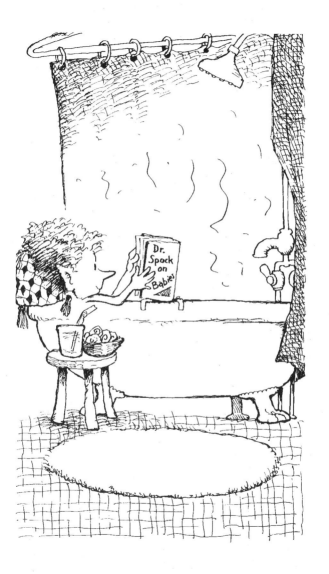

7.

Accept feelings of desperation and discouragement. Your life is changing completely!

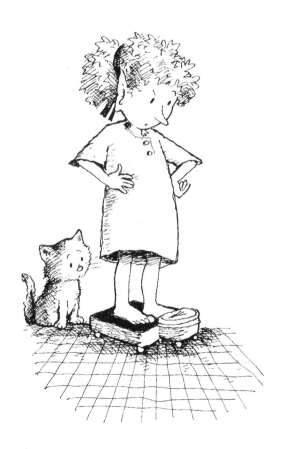

8.

Spend time with loved ones
now. Soon your child will
need most of your time.

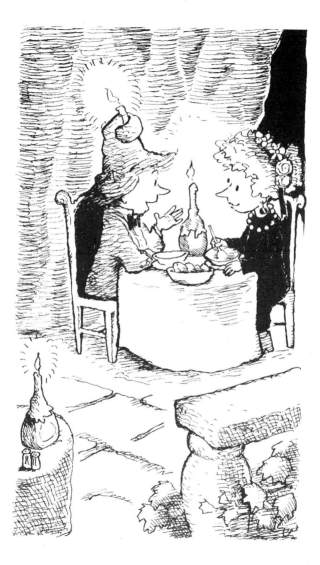

9.

Make plans for your future now. Build dreams for your family!

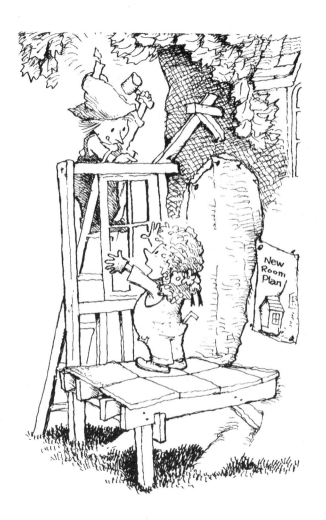

New
Room
Plan

10.

Reconsider present responsibilities. Bringing a child into the world is now your most important task.

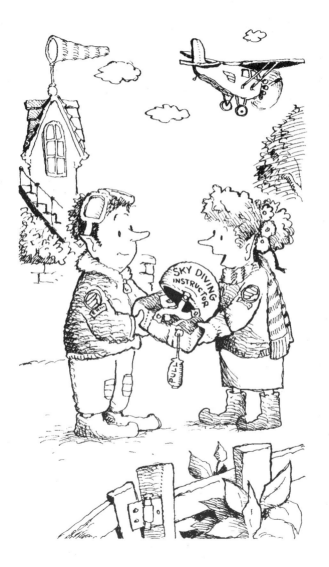

11.

Seek balance in your daily life. Play, dance, go for a walk!

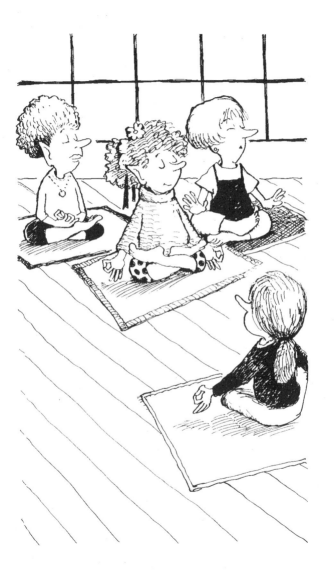

12.

Trust your intuition.
You know what is best
for you and your child.

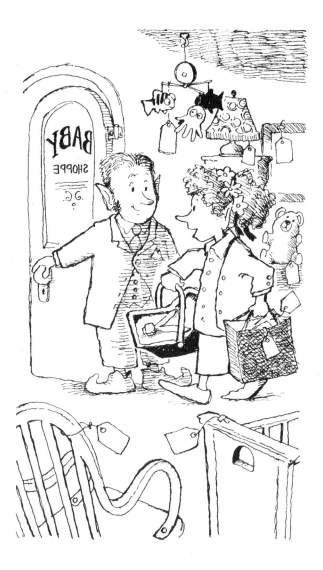

13.

Let others take care of you.
Caring for a woman who
is pregnant gives others
respect for life itself.

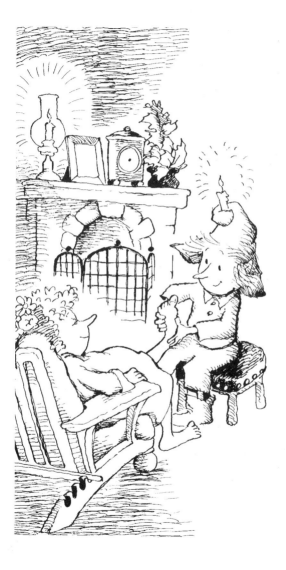

14.

Enjoy feeling one with your unborn child. You carry God's present to you.

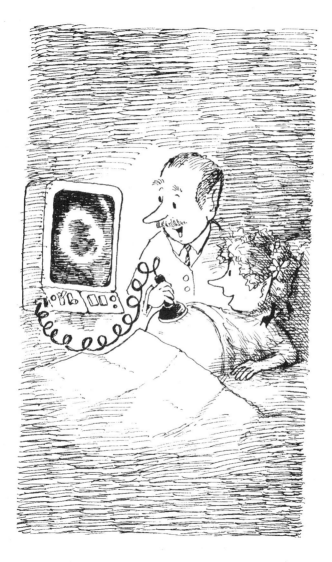

15.

Take care of yourself.
From you springs new life.

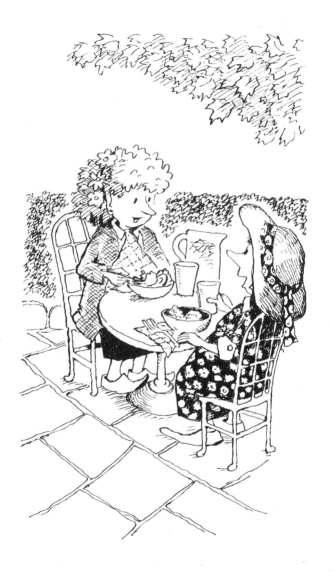

16.

Enjoy your pregnant body.
God's gift now transforms you.

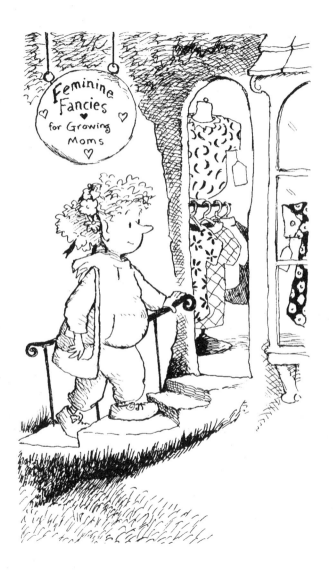

17.

Dress beautifully!
You look wonderful!

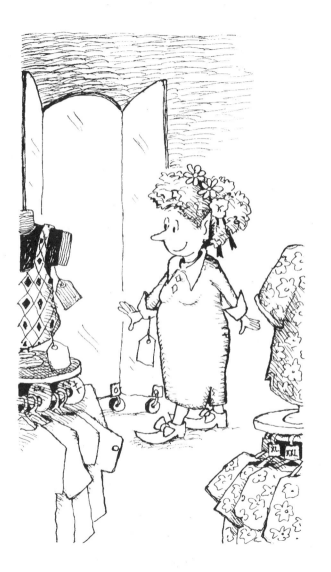

18.

Ask loved ones to share your daily chores. Even washing dishes can build togetherness.

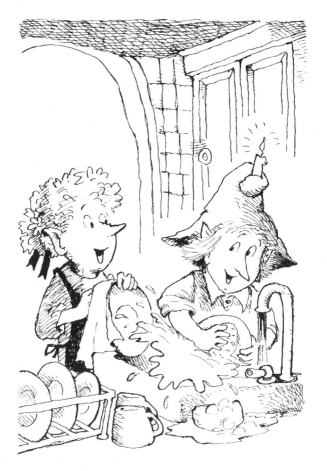

19.

Don't be frightened by thoughts of what could go wrong. Trust God's plans for you and your child.

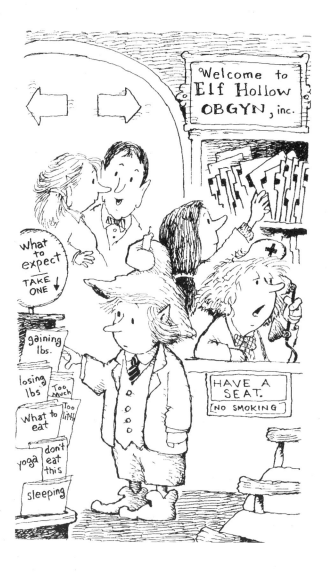

20.

Let yourself be inspired by
birds building nests and
nature's care for its young.

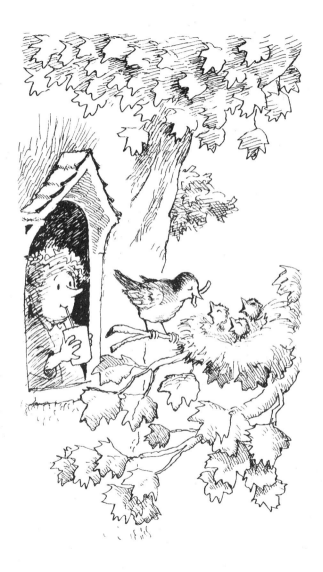

21.

If you have children already,
enjoy your time together now.
Strengthen the bonds that
connect you in your special
way forever.

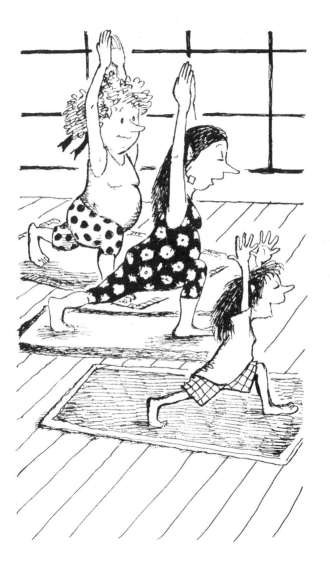

22.

Your love for your other children need not be divided. Mothers have plenty of love for all their children—born and unborn. In your heart, the love for your unborn child is growing like a beautiful flower.

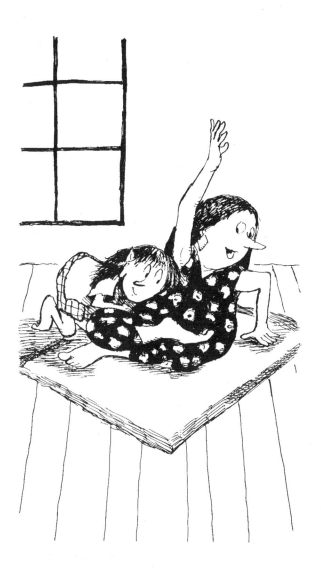

23.

Do not worry about how your
other children will cope with
your unborn child. They are
getting the sister or brother
God intends for them.

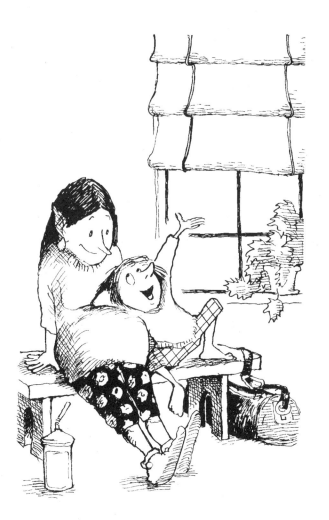

24.

Think lovingly of those who will not see the birth of your child. Your connection to them blesses you and your child.

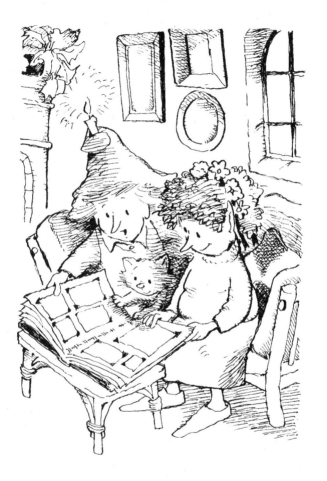

25.

Talk to your child. Get to know each other now.

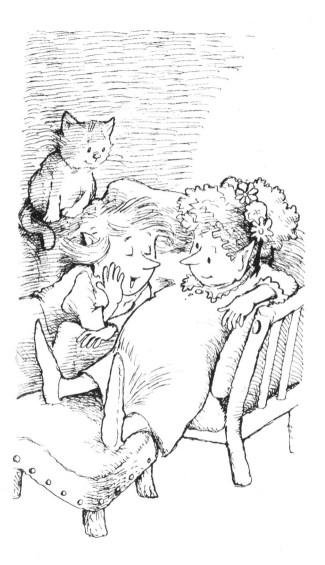

26.

Sing to your child. Music does the baby good.

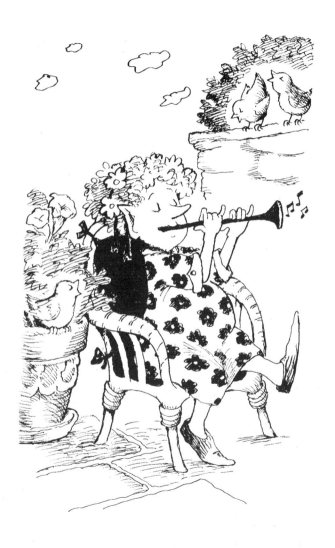

27.

Mothers-to-be need to be mothered! Provide yourself with motherly care.

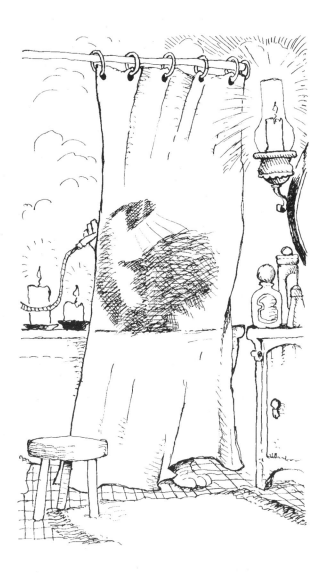

28.

You are going through times of insecurity and change. Look for pleasant and comfortable situations where you yourself have the feeling of being "carried."

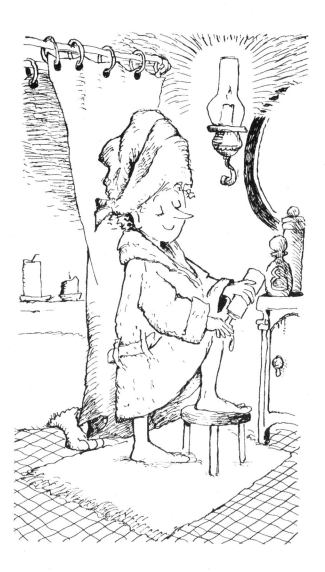

29.

Get together with other mothers-to-be. Shared experiences are a powerful means of support.

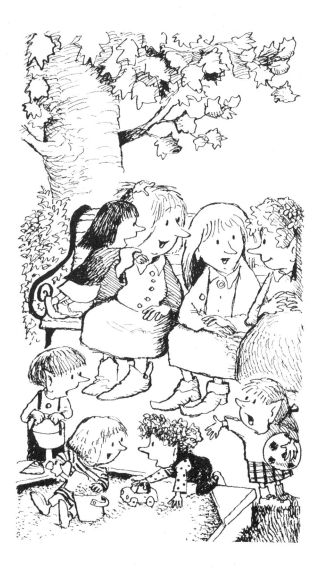

30.

Use your time of waiting
to prepare yourself—inside
and out.

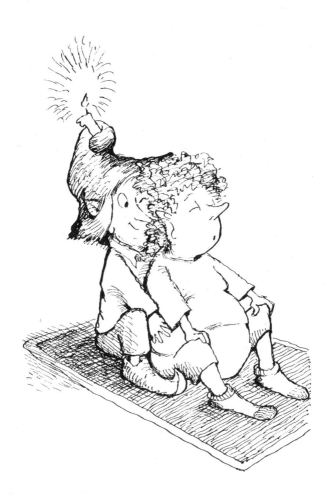

31.

Crying is normal. Tears soften your heart and prepare your soul for the arrival of your child.

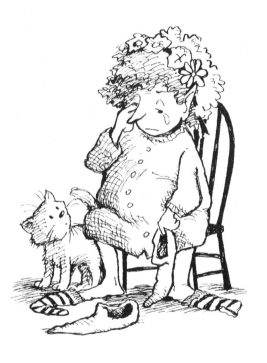

32.

Do what you enjoy now.
And trust that your new
life will provide many
future enjoyments.

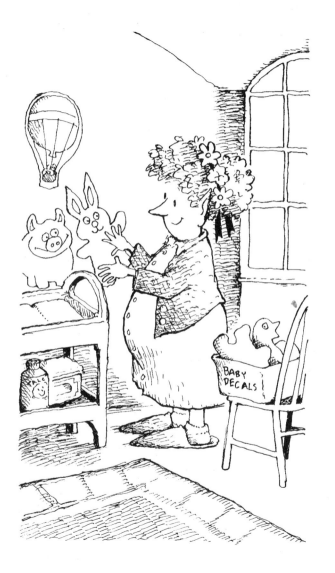

33.

If you lack the strength for everyday duties, let them go. Others will complete them.

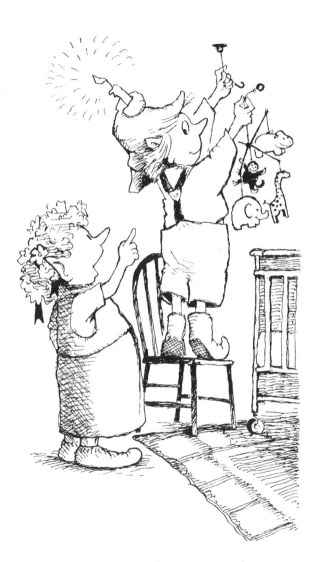

34.

When you doubt your abilities
as a mother, remember that
mothers are not perfect. Your
child will receive your best—
and your worst—and
everything in-between.

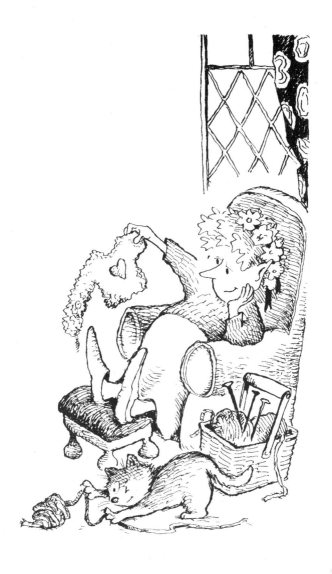

35.

Don't be afraid of giving birth. You have all that you need.

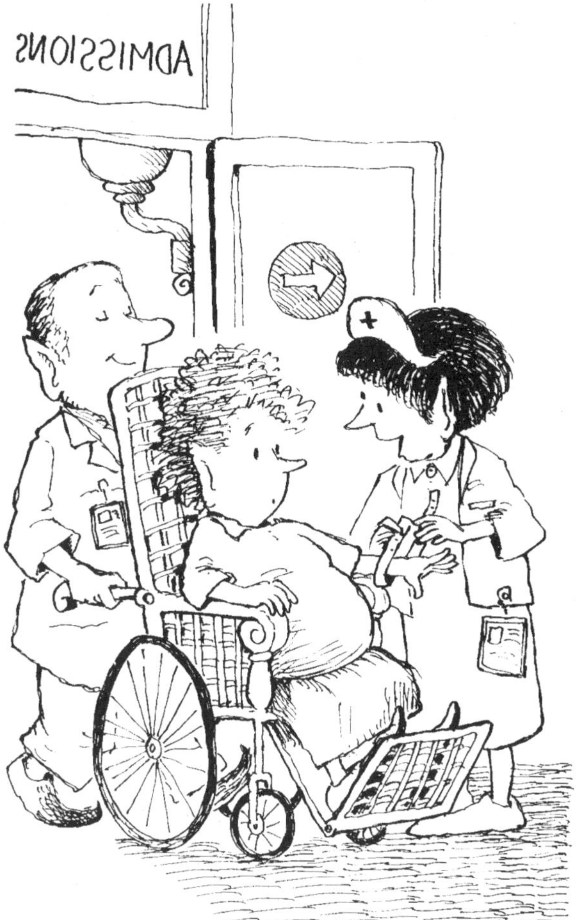
ADMISSIONS

36.

You are starting a new life and nobody can tell how it will be. Let yourself be guided by your courage, not by your fear!

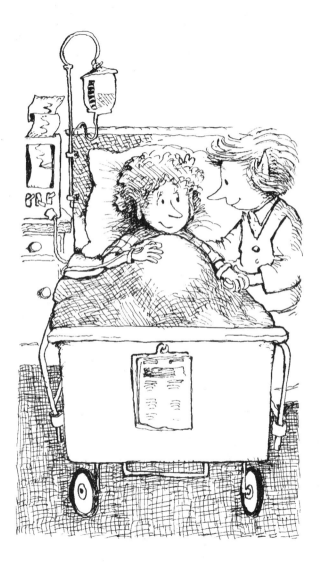

37.

When the moment comes for your child to be born, let it go! Your child does not belong to you, but to itself, to life, and to God.

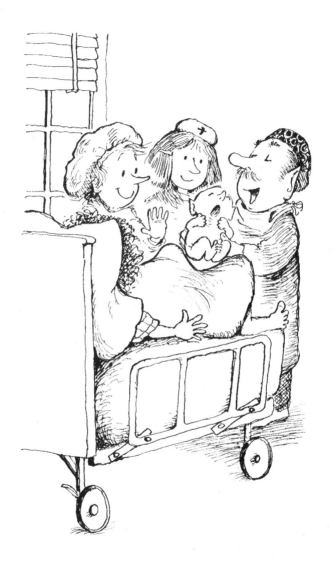

38.

Pray for your child.
God's ear is open to you.

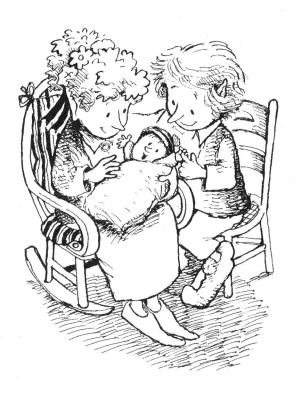

Claudia Bollwinkel conceived the idea for this book while pregnant with her second child. She works for the German Women's Foundation *filia die frauenstiftung*. She lives in Lüneburg, Germany, with her husband and two sons.

Illustrator for the Abbey Press Elf-help Books, **R.W. Alley**, also illustrates and writes children's books, including *Making a Boring Day Better—A Kid's Guide to Battling the Blahs*, a recent Elf-help Book for Kids.

The Story of the Abbey Press Elves

The engaging figures that populate the Abbey Press "elf-help" line of publications and products first appeared in 1987 on the pages of a small self-help book called *Be-good-to-yourself Therapy*. Shaped by the publishing staff's vision and defined in R.W. Alley's inventive illustrations, they lived out the author's gentle, self-nurturing advice with charm, poignancy, and humor.

Reader response was so enthusiastic that more Elf-help Books were soon under way, a still-growing series that has inspired a line of related gift products.

The especially endearing character featured in the early books—sporting a cap with a mood-changing candle in its peak—has since been joined by a spirited female elf with flowers in her hair.

These two exuberant, sensitive, resourceful, kindhearted, lovable sprites, along with their lively elfin community, reveal what's truly important as they offer messages of joy and wonder, playfulness and co-creation, wholeness and serenity, the miracle of life and the mystery of God's love.

With wisdom and whimsy, these little creatures with long noses demonstrate the elf-help way to a rich and fulfilling life.

Elf-help Books

...adding "a little character" and a lot
of help to self-help reading!

Elf-help for the Mother-to-Be	#20354
Believe-in-yourself Therapy	#20351
Grieving at Christmastime	#20052
Elf-help for Giving the Gift of You!	#20054
Grief Therapy (new, revised edition)	#20178
Healing Thoughts for Troubled Hearts	#20058
Take Charge of Your Eating	#20064
Elf-help for Coping With Pain	#20074
Elf-help for Dealing with Difficult People	#20076
Loneliness Therapy	#20078
Elf-help for Healing from Divorce	#20082
Music Therapy	#20083
'Tis a Blessing to Be Irish	#20088
Getting Older, Growing Wiser	#20089
Worry Therapy	#20093
Elf-help for Raising a Teen	#20102

Book price is $4.95 unless otherwise noted.
Available at your favorite gift shop or bookstore—
or directly from One Caring Place, Abbey Press
Publications, St. Meinrad, IN 47577.
Or call 1-800-325-2511.
www.carenotes.com